Hèla Ben Jmaà
Mariam Dammak
Sirine Frikha

Surgical treatment of atheromatous carotid stenosis

Hèla Ben Jmaà
Mariam Dammak
Sirine Frikha

Surgical treatment of atheromatous carotid stenosis

ScienciaScripts

Imprint

Any brand names and product names mentioned in this book are subject to trademark, brand or patent protection and are trademarks or registered trademarks of their respective holders. The use of brand names, product names, common names, trade names, product descriptions etc. even without a particular marking in this work is in no way to be construed to mean that such names may be regarded as unrestricted in respect of trademark and brand protection legislation and could thus be used by anyone.

Cover image: www.ingimage.com

This book is a translation from the original published under ISBN 978-620-6-71515-3.

Publisher:
Sciencia Scripts
is a trademark of
Dodo Books Indian Ocean Ltd. and OmniScriptum S.R.L publishing group

120 High Road, East Finchley, London, N2 9ED, United Kingdom
Str. Armeneasca 28/1, office 1, Chisinau MD-2012, Republic of Moldova, Europe
Printed at: see last page
ISBN: 978-620-7-78892-7

I- INTRODUCTION

Stroke is the leading cause of acquired disability in adults, and the second leading cause of death and dementia in Tunisia.

Knowledge of the pathophysiological mechanisms and main aetiologies of stroke is essential to ensure appropriate treatment.

Ischaemic strokes result from the obstruction of a cerebral artery by a blood clot and make up the majority of all strokes (around 87%) (1,2).

According to the ASCOD and TOAST classifications, atherosclerosis of the large arteries is one of the main causes of ischaemic stroke, with an estimated prevalence of 20%. Atheromatous lesions of arteries destined for the brain can progressively lead to haemodynamically significant stenosis, with the internal carotid artery and the carotid bifurcation being the preferred sites (3).

The therapeutic management of these atheromatous stenosing lesions is based on medical treatment, with or without surgical or endovascular treatment.

Carotid endarterectomy (CEA) currently remains the gold standard for revascularisation of the internal carotid artery (4).

The indications for carotid surgery depend on the degree of stenosis and whether or not the lesion is symptomatic, taking into account the results of randomised trials (NASCET, ACAS, ECST).

However, carotid surgery, which is essentially preventive in nature, is not without its risks of excess mortality and post-operative complications.

Current debates focus on the pre-operative assessment of patients, the choice of the appropriate surgical technique, and the close monitoring of patients during and after the operation.

II- EPIDEMIOLOGY

1- Frequency :

Table I: Number of carotid stenoses in the literature :

Authors	Workforce	Period
Archie (5)	1360	1983-1998
Ohara (6)	3360	1989-1999
P Garvin (7)	2331	2004-2017
M Meller (8)	718	2007-2013
J Sun (9)	547	2011-2017

2- Age and gender :

The predominance of males is highlighted by all the series in the literature. Symptomatic patients are predominantly male. On the other hand, females are more likely to be found in asymptomatic patients.

Table II: Population characteristics according to the literature :

Authors	Workforce	Average/median age	Percentage of men	Percentage of women
Archie (5)	1360	67 years old	56%	44%
P Garvin (3)	2331	70.7 years old	62,8%	37,2%
M Meller (8)	718	72 years old	62,2%	37,8%

3- Cardiovascular risk factors :

1- Hypertension :

High blood pressure (hypertension) is the most important cardiovascular risk factor.Atheromatous lesions are encouraged by poorly balanced blood pressure. Excessive blood pressure leads to thickening and hardening of the arteries, which contributes to the development of atherosclerosis, particularly in the arteries supplying the brain. According to the Framingham study (10), the risk of a stroke is 9-fold in men and 4-fold in women, in hypertensive patients. The risk of mortality is also high (11). Screening for and controlling hypertension is essential. New biomarkers are now available to predict the subsequent risk of developing atherosclerotic lesions in hypertensive patients, which could be a good marker for preventing carotid stenosis (12).

2- Diabetes :

Diabetes is a second major risk factor for atherosclerosis.

Chronic, poorly controlled diabetes contributes to the maintenance of atherogenesis through the glycation of lipoproteins (13). It would also appear that the adhesion of chemotactic and pro-inflammatory factors to endothelial cells is increased in diabetics. This explains the prevalence of atheromatous lesions in this category of patients. Cardiovascular mortality is also 4 times higher in diabetic patients than in non-diabetic patients (14). Strict control of diabetes and associated cardiovascular risk factors is essential to ensure better prevention.

3- Tobacco :

Smoking is a major public health problem. The cardio-vascular risk caused by smoking is proportional to the length of time you smoke and the amount you smoke each day.Smoking is associated with changes in lipid levels, reduced fibrinolysis and changes in endothelial and platelet structures (15).

4- Dyslipidemia :

Underlying dyslipidaemia is considered to be a major risk factor for cardiovascular disease.Hyperlipidaemia plays an important role in the maintenance of oxidative stress, inflammation and endothelial dysfunction. (16) In carotid pathology, it is above all total cholesterol and HDL-cholesterol levels that contribute to the maintenance of atherosclerosis in cerebral arteries (17).

III-CLINICAL MANIFESTATIONS OF CAROTID STENOSIS: 1-CIRCUMSTANCES OF DISCOVERY

1- Symptomatic patients :

Symptomatic stenosis is associated with a significant risk of stroke. This risk is particularly high in the days or weeks following the first infarction (18).

It is important to identify the circumstances in which symptomatic carotid stenosis develops, in order to guide the diagnostic and therapeutic course of action. Symptoms may be neurological, suggesting a diagnosis of ischaemic stroke or transient ischaemic attack (TIA) systematised in the carotid territory. Symptoms may be isolated or associated, resulting in a clinical polymorphism. The attribution of these neurological events to atherosclerosis is more strongly suggested if the subject is elderly and in the presence of one or more cardiovascular risk factors.Any other non-specific symptomatology would classify the patient as asymptomatic.

2- Asymptomatic patients :

This group includes patients with no neurological symptoms suggestive of a carotid stroke, or with clinical symptoms suggesting neurological damage suggestive of a vertebro-basilar territory (headache, vertigo, vomiting, etc.).

The prevalence of asymptomatic carotid stenosis is only very imperfectly known. The increase in this prevalence is conditioned by the presence of cardiovascular risk factors and other atheromatous locations (19).

A study by Pujia A et al (20), including apparently healthy patients from the general population, showed that the prevalence and severity of carotid disease increased with age, particularly between the decades [65-74] and [75-84].

Current recommendations from the European Society of Cardiology (ESC) advise against systematic screening for asymptomatic carotid lesions in the general population (21).

This approach is of interest in patients with multiple cardiovascular risk factors, in order to reduce the subsequent risk of morbidity and mortality. In France, screening is mainly recommended for patients with coronary artery disease or obliterative arterial disease of the lower limbs (22). In current practice, exploration of the carotid arteries in an asymptomatic patient with cardiovascular risk factors is recommended in three essential circumstances:

✓ Systematic screening of patients with arterial disease or coronary heart disease.

✓ Clinical examination reveals a cervical murmur.

✓ Preoperative assessment for open-heart surgery.

2- Clinical examination :

The clinical assessment of patients with carotid stenosis, particularly in the cardiovascular and neurological fields, is essential.

Carotid murmurs are important to look for on examination. Its presence is correlated with the existence of carotid stenosis, without prejudging its severity (23). Heart murmurs should also be sought, as they may indicate an underlying cardiac pathology. The neurological examination is part of the pre-operative assessment of patients. The presence of neurological deficits is an indication of the topography and extent of the ischaemic lesions.

IV- ASSESSMENT OF CAROTID STENOSIS

At the end of the epidemiological and clinical investigation, the suspicion of a carotid stenosis of atherosclerotic origin requires additional examinations.

Once the gold standard, invasive angiography of the carotid arteries is now being abandoned in favour of the development of new equipment and techniques.

Non-invasive vascular imaging has played an important role in recent years, making it possible to study the quality of the carotid arteries and estimate the degree of stenosis.

1- Doppler ultrasound of the supra-aortic trunks :

Doppler ultrasound of the supra-aortic trunks (AST) is a simple, inexpensive and reproducible test. Its ease of access and simplicity mean that it is widely used as a first-line examination. This is the only test that provides both morphological and velocimetric data (24). Doppler ultrasound can be used to study the morphology of the plaque responsible for the stenosis and the quality of the walls upstream and downstream of the stenosis.The morphological description of the plaque echostructure includes: echogenicity, texture, size and surface.

The velocimetric study or velocity analysis is based on recording peak peak velocity and end-diastolic velocity at the site of stenosis in each artery, including both internal, external and common carotid arteries. A peak systolic velocity greater than 200 cm per second generally indicates a stenosis of 50% or more (23). The combination of morphological and velocimetric data makes it possible to quantify internal carotid artery stenoses and assess their impact (25) (Figures 1 and 2).

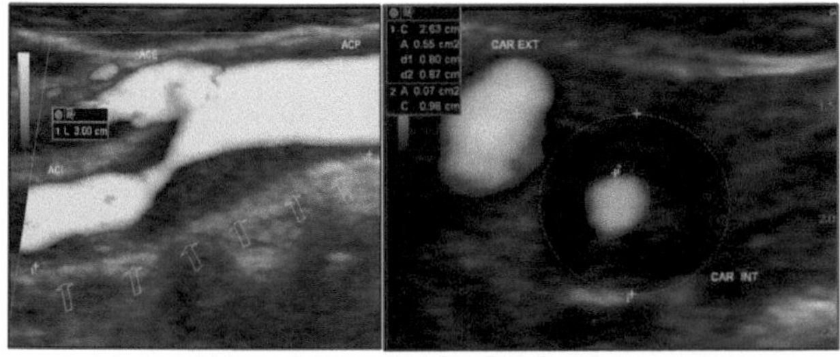

Figures 1 and 2: Visualisation of a narrowing of the internal carotid artery on Doppler ultrasound.

Doppler ultrasound of ASD is estimated to have a sensitivity of between 90 and 95%, with a specificity of between 80 and 96% (26).

Post-operatively, Doppler ultrasound is also the examination of choice for monitoring and radiological surveillance of the risk of thrombosis or atheromatous restenosis of the operated internal carotid artery and the contralateral artery.

The limits of this examination are its operator-dependent nature, the existence of arterial calcifications, loops, plicatures and high situated bulbs which can constitute a shadow zone on ultrasound and hinder visualisation of the arterial lumen. Doppler ultrasound of the supra-aortic trunks does not allow exploration of the intracranial axes. Some teams supplement ultrasound exploration with trans-cranial Doppler ultrasound, which allows assessment of the downstream impact of extra-cranial carotid stenosis and evaluation of the quality of intracranial bypass (27).

At present, it would be advisable to carry out two explorations of the supra-aortic trunks, with congruent results, before any surgical or endovascular intervention for carotid stenosis. Some studies suggest that Doppler ultrasound should be one of the mandatory examinations among the two mentioned above (28).

2- Helical angioscan of the supra-aortic trunks :

Helical angioscanner is a non-invasive and reliable technique, offering three-dimensional reconstruction of the carotid axes, a study of the arterial lumen and wall, and atherosclerotic plaque (29). Angioscan is considered to be the examination of choice. It has the advantage of providing the best possible view of the carotid bifurcation. The diagnosis of pseudo-occlusive stenosis appears to be particularly reliable with this technique (22).The results of angioscan are consistent with intra-arterial angiography in over 90% of cases (30). Its sensitivity for assessing the degree of stenosis varies from 70 to 100% and its specificity varies from 95 to 100%, for stenoses greater than 70% (31) (Figure 3).

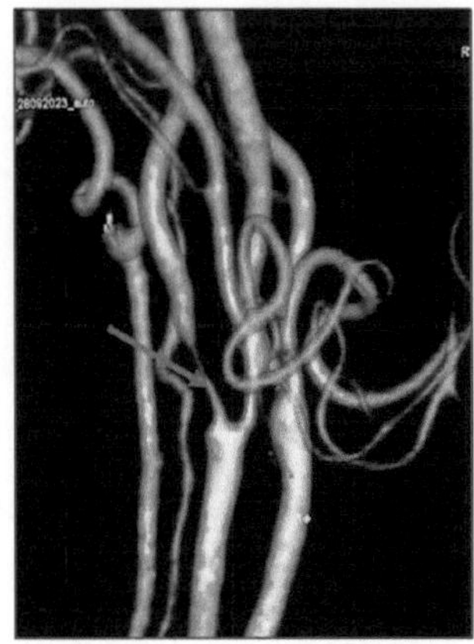

Figure 3: Hyper-tight stenosis of the right internal carotid artery.

Furthermore, the information gathered during this examination is morphological and not dynamic, making it impossible to study arterial flow. The existence of arterial calcifications is also a limitation of this examination, making analysis of the contact lumen difficult (32). It should not be used on patients with acute or chronic renal failure, or who are allergic to the contrast medium.

3- Magnetic resonance angiography (MRA) :

Magnetic resonance angiography offers the advantage of visualising the atheromatous lesion, the arterial tree, both extra- and intracranial, in its entirety, as well as the state of the cerebral parenchyma with much greater precision than is possible with cerebral CT. Detailed analysis of the characteristics of the carotid plaque is also possible using magnetic resonance imaging (Figure 4).

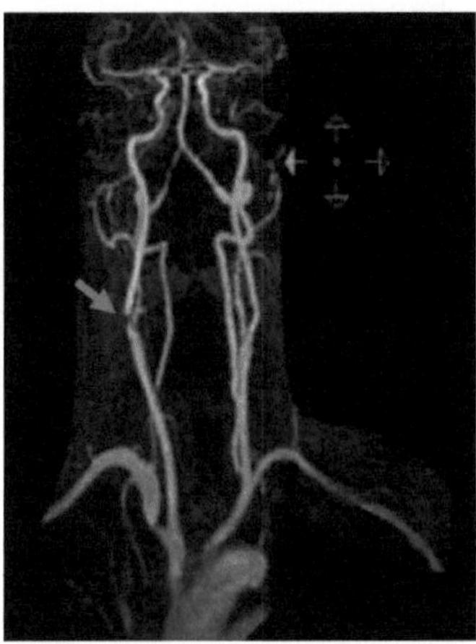

Figure 4: Three-dimensional reconstruction of the supra-aortic trunks showing stenosis of the right carotid bulb (arrow) (33).

Severe stenoses (>70%) are detected with a sensitivity and specificity of over 85% when this test is performed alone, and with a sensitivity and specificity of over 95% when it is combined with Doppler ultrasound (34).

Studies have compared the results of MRA with the pathological analysis of endarterectomy specimens and have shown the reliability of this examination in the study of the fibrous and lipid component of the plaque and in the detection of intra-plate haemorrhagic zones, which are considered to be criteria for assessing the risk of embolism of the carotid lesion. Of course, this depends on the performance of the MRI scanners available, which are not all equally effective in all centres (35). However, the limitations of MRA essentially come down to its tendency to overestimate the degree of stenosis, which could lead to two types of error

: (36, 37).

- Or consider that a stenosis is potentially operable when its actual degree is below the accepted threshold for intervention.

- Or make the diagnosis of occlusion when there is a pseudo-occlusive stenosis with very slow downstream flow (Figure 5).

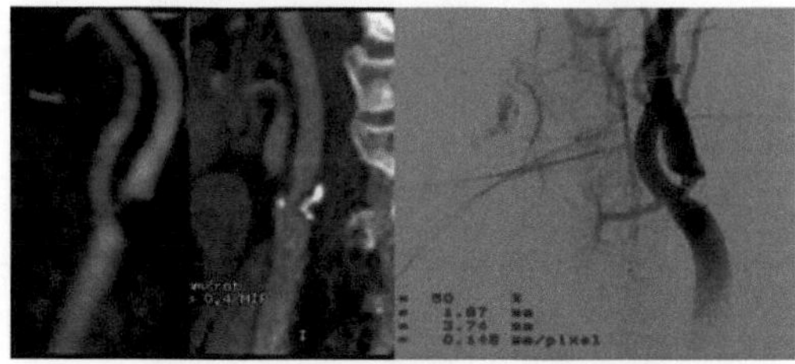

Figure 5: Example of overestimation of ASD in MRA of a carotid bifurcation stenosis, overestimated by more than 70%, and actually measuring 50% on angiography-CT and arteriography (37).

Contraindications (Pacemaker, claustrophobia, metallic foreign body, etc.) may also limit its use.

4- Arteriography of the supra-aortic trunks :

This examination, which used to be the Gold Standard, enables the vessels destined for the brain to be studied from the aortic arch to the terminal intracranial branches, collateral circulation to be assessed, and the appearance of the atheromatous plaque and the regularity of its surface to be evaluated (33) (Figure 6).

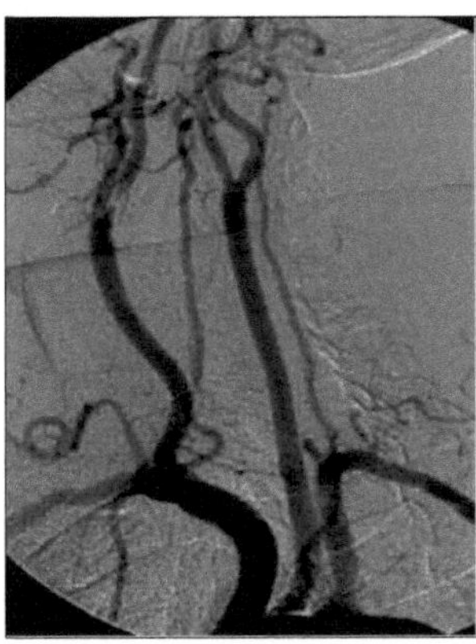

Figure 6: Angiography of the supra-aortic trunks showing tight calcified stenosis of the origin of the right internal carotid artery (arrow) (33).

In the two large randomised studies (NASCET and ECST), angiography made an essential contribution to quantifying the degree of carotid stenosis by analysing two perpendicular views.

The stenosis was quantified on angiography, in the incidence where it was tightest. The diameter of the circulating channel was related to two denominators: the diameter of the healthy internal carotid artery downstream of the stenosis for the American method (38), and the total carotid bulb obtained by reconstruction for the European method (39) (Figure 7).

It follows that the stenoses included in NASCET were anatomically less tight than those included in ECST: a 70% stenosis in NASCET corresponded to approximately 82% in ECST. Currently, the recommended quantification for the assessment of carotid stenosis is NASCET quantification (40).

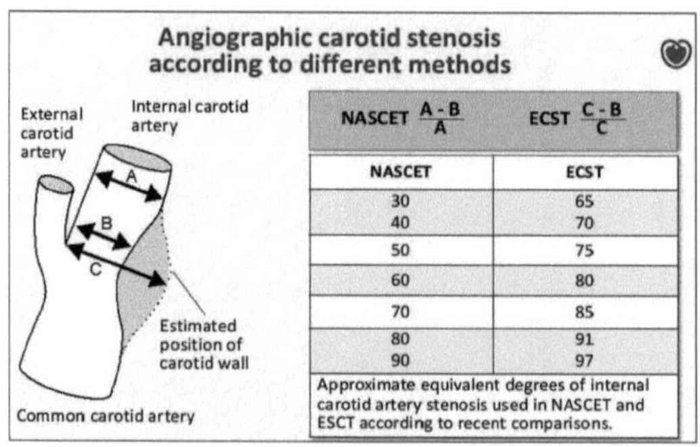

NASCET	ECST
30	65
40	70
50	75
60	80
70	85
80	91
90	97
Approximate equivalent degrees of internal carotid artery stenosis used in NASCET and ESCT according to recent comparisons.	

Figure 7: Assessment of degrees of stenosis based on angiography according to NASCET and ECST (40).

The disadvantages of angiography, which have limited its use in recent years, are its invasive nature, which exposes patients to a high risk of vascular complications linked in particular to the arterial puncture zone (bleeding, haematoma, acute ischaemia), and neurological complications linked to the migration of calcareous emboli. Neurological complications were demonstrated in the ACAS study, where the rate of these complications was high at 1.2%, i.e. half the cumulative 30-day morbidity and mortality rate (2.3%) (41). The use of this technique in patients who are being considered for surgery could therefore lead to a further increase in intra- and post-operative mortality.

5- Brain imaging :

Cerebral imaging using CT or MRI is a fundamental examination for assessing the cerebral parenchyma. It should be performed systematically whenever there is a suspicion of stroke.Cerebral imaging confirms the presence of a stroke, specifying whether it is ischaemic or haemorrhagic and the area of the brain affected. It can also be used to estimate the extent and severity of the lesions. Cerebral imaging is preferred in symptomatic patients with a suggestive neurological picture. Some teams systematically perform preoperative brain scans, in asymptomatic patients, to detect silent brain lesions (42).

V-INDICATIONS FOR CAROTID ENDARTERECTOMY

The role of carotid endarterectomy in the management of atheromatous stenosis has been well codified. It consists of preventing the risk of subsequent cerebral infarction in cases of significant carotid stenosis (43).Efficient and optimal revascularisation of carotid stenosis reduces the risk of stroke in asymptomatic patients in primary prevention and symptomatic patients in secondary prevention.Over the years, a number of randomised studies have been carried out to assess the benefit of carotid surgery. These studies compared, after randomisation, the risk of neurological events and/or death in patients with carotid stenosis, treated either by medical treatment alone or by medical treatment combined with surgical treatment. Various studies have concluded that surgical treatment, combined with well-managed medical treatment, is of paramount importance.

1- Symptomatic patients :

1- NASCET study (North American Symptomatic Carotid Endarterectomy) : In the American NASCET study (44), symptomatic patients aged less than 80 years were included who had suffered a hemispheric or retinal ischaemic stroke within the previous 120 days in association with homolateral carotid stenosis of a degree of between 30 and 99%.Patients with homolateral carotid siphon stenosis of a degree greater than or equal to proximal stenosis and patients at high surgical risk were excluded from this study. The surgical teams taking part in the study were selected on the basis of a cumulative morbidity-mortality rate of less than 6%. Randomisation involved either surgery combined with medical treatment (surgical group) or medical treatment alone (medical group). The results of the study were as follows:

✓ For stenoses ≥ 70% :

o The results at two years for the 659 patients showed that the cumulative rate of ipsilateral stroke was 26% in the medical group compared with 9% in the surgical group (P<0.001), corresponding to a reduction in the risk of stroke at 2 years of 17% in absolute terms and 65% in relative terms (39).

o Overall mortality was 5.5%, 6.3% in the non-operated group and 4.6% in the operated group. The difference was not significant.

✓ For stenoses between 50 and 69% :

o The results of the NASCET study published at 5 years (44) showed that surgery was of no benefit for certain sub-groups, in particular women and retinal signs.

o The rate of homolateral stroke after 5 years' follow-up was 15.7% in the surgical group compared with 22.2% in the medical group.

✓ For stenoses <50%: the results of the two groups were equivalent. 2- European Carotid Surgery Trial (ECST):
The European study included symptomatic patients with hemispheric or retinal ischemic stroke, with no age limit. The ischaemic event was less than 6 months old and related to a homolateral carotid stenosis of 99% or less (45, 46).

Randomisation involved either surgery combined with medical treatment or medical treatment alone. Any post-operative stroke lasting more than 7 days was taken into account.

The results of this study showed :

✓ For stenoses ≥ 70% (39):

o The cumulative rate of homolateral stroke at 3 years was 16.8% in the medical group and 2.8% in the surgical group. The reduction in absolute risk was therefore 14% and in relative risk 85%.

o The combined reduction in the risk of stroke and post-operative death was 6.5% as an absolute risk and 39% as a relative risk in the surgical group compared with the medical group.

o The difference in overall mortality between the two groups was not significant.

✓ For stenoses between 30 and 69% (39, 46):

o The overall survival rate was not statistically different between the surgical and medical groups.

✓ For stenoses < 30% (45) :

o The rate of stroke was 0.4% per year. The risk of death and post-operative stroke was 4.6%, and there was no significant difference in the overall mortality rate between the surgical group and the medical group. There was therefore no benefit from surgery.

In terms of time to onset of vascular events, the risk of death or major stroke was statistically higher: (45)

✓ During the period between 0 and 2.3 years of follow-up, for stenoses between 50 and 69%.

✓ During the period between 0 and 3.4 years of follow-up, for stenoses between 30 and 49%.

✓ Beyond these follow-up times, the risk of death or stroke did not differ significantly between the medical and surgical groups, whatever the degree of stenosis.

2- Asymptomatic patients :

1- ACAS (Asymptomatic Carotid Atherosclerosis Study) :

The ACAS study (47) included patients aged between 40 and 79, at low surgical risk, and with stenoses ≥ 60%.These patients were randomised into two groups:

a medical group and a surgical group. Degrees of stenosis were measured by Doppler ultrasound and plethysmography. Angiography was performed only in the surgical group. The peri-operative morbidity and mortality rate was 2.3%, including complications of arteriography (1.2%). Morbidity and mortality were significantly higher in cases of previous ischaemic stroke or contralateral stenosis of more than 60%.

The 5-year results showed that :

✓ The risk of cerebral infarction homolateral to the stenosis was 2.2% per year.

✓ The risk of stroke and death was 11% in the medical group, compared with 5.1% in the surgical group.

✓ The relative risk reduction was 53% and the absolute risk reduction was 5.9%, or 1.2% per year.

✓ The benefit of surgery did not become apparent until 3 years after the operation. This benefit did not increase with the degree of stenosis.

✓ The benefit of surgery was not significant for disabling strokes or for mortality. It was significant for all TIAs and homolateral infarctions.

2- ACST (Asymptomatic Carotid Surgery Trial) :

This study (48) included patients who had been asymptomatic for at least 6 months and had carotid stenoses $\geq$ 60% diagnosed by Doppler ultrasound. Patients with a history of homolateral endarterectomy, those with a high operative risk in relation to recent MI or embologenic heart disease, and those with another major threatening comorbidity were excluded. Patients were classified into four groups, according to the degree of stenosis established by Doppler ultrasound: 60%, 70%, 80% and 90%. Angiography was not required. This study showed that :

✓ The risk of stroke was 6% in the immediate endarterectomy group compared with 12% in the delayed endarterectomy group.

✓ The benefit of surgery was that disabling strokes were halved.

✓ The benefit was significant for both men and women under the age of 65, and between 65 and 74 for stenoses of 70%, 80% and 90% (48).

This study therefore confirms the benefit of carotid surgery for asymptomatic stenoses of over 70%, combined with optimised treatment of vascular risk factors.

3- Current indications for carotid endarterectomy :

Several recommendations with a high level of evidence have been proposed by learned authorities, including: American Heart Association, American Stroke Association (2006), Haute Autorité de Santé Française (2007), European Society for Vascular Surgery (2009) and American Academy of Neurology (2013).

The latest recommendations, currently established, were recorded in 2017 by the European Society of Cardiology (ESC), in collaboration with the European Society for Vascular Surgery (ESVS).

The 2017 ESC recommendations state that: (Figures 8 and 9)

✓ For **asymptomatic** patients :

o Carotid endarterectomy is recommended in patients presenting an average surgical risk with a degree of stenosis between 60

and 99% and in the presence of clinical and/or radiological features associated with a significant risk of ischaemic stroke ipsilateral to the stenosis, provided that the patient's life expectancy exceeds 5 years and the risk of stroke or death at 30 days is <3%.

o If there is a high surgical risk, a carotid stent is the ideal solution.

Recommendations for management of asymptomatic carotid artery disease

Recommendations	Class[a]	Level[b]
In 'average surgical risk' patients with an asymptomatic 60–99% stenosis, CEA should be considered in the presence of clinical and/or more imaging characteristics[c] that may be associated with an increased risk of late ipsilateral stroke, provided documented perioperative stroke/death rates are <3% and the patient's life expectancy is > 5 years.[116]	IIa	B
In asymptomatic patients who have been deemed 'high risk for CEA'[d] and who have an asymptomatic 60–99% stenosis in the presence of clinical and/or imaging characteristics[c] that may be associated with an increased risk of late ipsilateral stroke, CAS should be considered, provided documented perioperative stroke/death rates are <3% and the patient's life expectancy is > 5 years.[135,136]	IIa	B
In 'average surgical risk' patients with an asymptomatic 60–99% stenosis in the presence of clinical and/or imaging characteristics[d] that may be associated with an increased risk of late ipsilateral stroke, CAS may be an alternative to CEA provided documented perioperative stroke/death rates are <3% and the patient's life expectancy is > 5 years.[110,129,132,137]	IIb	B

BP = blood pressure, CAS = carotid artery stenting, CEA = carotid endarterectomy.
[a]Class of recommendation.
[b]Level of evidence.
[c]See *Table 4* and Web Table 5.
[d]Age >80 years, clinically significant cardiac disease, severe pulmonary disease, contralateral internal carotid artery occlusion, contralateral recurrent laryngeal nerve palsy, previous radical neck surgery or radiotherapy and recurrent stenosis after CEA.

Figure 8: European recommendations for revascularisation of asymptomatic carotid stenosis (21).

✓ For **symptomatic** patients:

o In case of stenosis between 70 and 99%, carotid endarterectomy is recommended, provided that the risk of morbidity and mortality is low.<6%.

o In the case of stenosis between 50 and 69%, endarterectomy should be considered if the risk of morbidity and mortality is < 6%.

o In cases of stenosis of between 50 and 99% associated with a high surgical risk, carotid stenting is recommended if the risk of morbidity and mortality is

< 6%.

o In the case of an average surgical risk, a carotid stent may be considered if the risk of morbidity and mortality is < 6%.

o Revascularisation is not recommended if the stenosis is <50%.

Recommendations on revascularization in patients with symptomatic carotid disease*

Recommendations	Class[a]	Level[b]
CEA is recommended in symptomatic patients with 70–99% carotid stenoses, provided the documented procedural death/stroke rate is < 6%.[138,147]	I	A
CEA should be considered in symptomatic patients with 50–69% carotid stenoses, provided the documented procedural death/stroke rate is < 6%.[138,147]	IIa	A
In recently symptomatic patients with a 50–99% stenosis who present with adverse anatomical features or medical comorbidities that are considered to make them 'high risk for CEA', CAS should be considered, provided the documented procedural death/stroke rate is < 6%.[135,145,152]	IIa	B
When revascularization is indicated in 'average surgical risk' patients with symptomatic carotid disease, CAS may be considered as an alternative to surgery, provided the documented procedural death/stroke rate is < 6%.[152,153]	IIb	B
When decided, it is recommended to perform revascularization of symptomatic 50–99% carotid stenoses as soon as possible, preferably within 14 days of symptom onset.[138,154,155]	I	A
Revascularization is not recommended in patients with a < 50% carotid stenosis.[138]	III	A

*Stroke or TIA occurring within 6 months.

Figure 9: European recommendations for revascularisation of symptomatic carotid stenosis (21).

VI- TIME TO ENDARTERECTOMY

There are three possible scenarios:

- Surgery for symptomatic patients.

- Surgery in asymptomatic patients.

- Surgery in cases of bilateral carotid involvement.

1- In symptomatic patients :

According to American and European recommendations, the ultimate risk of a constitutive ischaemic stroke is greatest in the 15 days following the first ischaemic episode in patients with carotid stenosis (49, 50).

Several reviews based on the NASCET and ECST data (51, 52) have shown that in these two large studies, in patients operated on at varying times from the onset of the last symptoms, carotid surgery was beneficial if performed within two weeks of the neurological event. This hypothesis was initially controversial.Indeed, some studies (52) have concluded, by comparing groups of patients operated on at varying times, that the best surgical delay would be equal to four weeks following the neurological event.Another study by Fairhead JF et al (53), based on NASCET data, showed that early surgery in patients with severe stenosis and non-disabling stroke had the same risk of death and major stroke post-operatively as late surgery. According to the latest ESC 2017 recommendations (21), endarterectomy should be performed within a maximum of 2 weeks of the ischaemic event, in symptomatic patients (Figure 10).

Recommendation 40	Class	Level
When revascularisation is considered appropriate in symptomatic patients with 50–99% stenoses, it is recommended that this be performed as soon as possible, preferably within 14 days of symptom onset	I	A
Recommendation 41		
Patients who are to undergo revascularisation within the first 14 days after onset of symptoms should undergo carotid endarterectomy, rather than carotid stenting	I	A

Figure 10: Time to carotid endarterectomy according to European recommendations (21).

Surgery could be carried out at a later date in three cases, in patients :

✓ Suffering from a disabling stroke with a modified Rankin score >=3.

✓ Presenting a severe disorder of consciousness.

✓ If brain imaging shows an extensive stroke (greater than 30% of the territory of the middle cerebral artery) or cerebral haemorrhage.

In these cases, it would be preferable to operate on patients within 6 to 8 weeks, given the considerable risk of haemorrhagic transformation (54) (Figure 11).

Recommendation 42	Class	Level
Revascularisation should be deferred in patients with 50–99% stenoses who suffer a disabling stroke (modified Rankin score $\geq$3), whose area of infarction exceeds one-third of the ipsilateral middle cerebral artery territory, or who have altered consciousness/ drowsiness, to minimise the risks of postoperative parenchymal haemorrhage	I	C

Figure 11: European recommendations concerning the time to intervention in cases of extensive stroke (21).

Furthermore, for patients with carotid stenosis >50% and multiple or crescendoing transient ischaemic attacks, surgery should be performed as a matter of urgency within 24 hours (Figure 12).

Recommendation 43		
Patients with 50–99% stenoses who present with stroke-in-evolution or crescendo transient ischaemic attacks should be considered for urgent carotid endarterectomy, preferably <24 hours	IIa	C

Figure 12: European recommendations for carotid revascularisation in transient ischaemic attacks (21).

2- In asymptomatic patients :

Carotid surgery in asymptomatic patients does not require the same emergency or semi-emergency management as for symptomatic patients, since the relationship between the degree of stenosis and the risk of homolateral cerebral infarction is relatively weak and there is no specific time limit to be respected (21).

3- Surgery in cases of bilateral carotid involvement :

This clinical situation occurs most frequently in a symptomatic or asymptomatic patient, in whom exploration of the supra-aortic trunks reveals a significant ipsilateral stenosis associated with an asymptomatic contralateral stenosis. The association of two symptomatic carotid stenoses is very rare. The interval between two operations for bilateral internal carotid stenosis is three weeks, in order to avoid hypertensive flare-ups that may be related to damage to the efferent nerves of the carotid sinus during the first operation.

VII- MEDICAL TREATMENT

Several trials have shown that low-dose anti-platelet agents (80-325mg/day), started pre-operatively, reduce the risk of neurological and coronary events at best, without increasing the risk of death. bleeding morbidity of the procedure. In a randomised, double-blind, placebo-controlled study, Lindblad et al (55) found that :

✓ The cumulative rate of major stroke and death at 30 days was 0.8% in patients treated with aspirin 75 mg/day pre-operatively, compared with 10.4% in patients treated with placebo (p<0.001).

✓ Intra-operative bleeding and re-operations for haemorrhage did not differ between the two groups.

According to the 2017 ESC recommendations: (21)
✓ Control of cardiovascular risk factors and blood pressure is recommended both pre-operatively and intraoperatively, with appropriate medical treatment.

✓ Simple platelet anti-aggregation with aspirin or clopidogrel is recommended in patients undergoing carotid surgery. Double anti-aggregation is recommended for patients undergoing stenting.

Figure 13 illustrates the treatment plan.

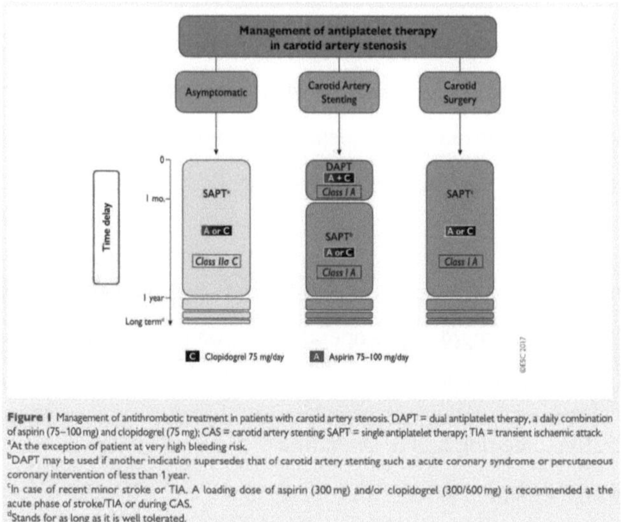

Figure I Management of antithrombotic treatment in patients with carotid artery stenosis. DAPT = dual antiplatelet therapy, a daily combination of aspirin (75–100 mg) and clopidogrel (75 mg); CAS = carotid artery stenting; SAPT = single antiplatelet therapy; TIA = transient ischaemic attack.
[a]At the exception of patient at very high bleeding risk.
[b]DAPT may be used if another indication supersedes that of carotid artery stenting such as acute coronary syndrome or percutaneous coronary intervention of less than 1 year.
[c]In case of recent minor stroke or TIA. A loading dose of aspirin (300 mg) and/or clopidogrel (300/600 mg) is recommended at the acute phase of stroke/TIA or during CAS.
[d]Stands for as long as it is well tolerated.

Figure 13: European anti-aggregation recommendations platelets (21).

VIII- PRE-OPERATIVE ASSESSMENT

1- Cardiovascular assessment and preparation :

The aim of this assessment is to identify patients with unbalanced hypertension or advanced ischaemic heart disease:

✓ Preoperative blood pressure monitoring is essential to reduce the risk of high blood pressure and/or neurological events.

✓ According to the new recommendations, screening for coronary artery disease, including coronary angiography, is recommended (21).

2- Neurological risk assessment :

One of the major complications of carotid surgery is the risk of neurological vascular accident. The latter may be caused by carotid clamping during the operation, which results in a hypo-flow in the downstream hemisphere, the extent and impact of which are variable, depending on the collateral circulation supplied by the other pedicles and above all by the polygon of Willis. Other risk factors are also associated with an increase in neurological morbidity, such as preoperative neurological instability and the absence of effective bypass surgery.For this reason, exploration of the supra-aortic trunks should be coupled, at best, with exploration by trans-cranial Doppler or MRI angiography, which allow assessment of the effectiveness of the supplements useful during carotid clamping (56).

IX- TYPES OF ANAESTHESIA

1- Preparing the patient :

Blood pressure is monitored continuously by invasive blood pressure measurement.Oxygen saturation is measured by percutaneous oximetry using a sensor placed on the patient's finger. Capnia is measured by a capnometer integrated into the artificial ventilation device. An electrocardiogram is essential for detecting myocardial ischaemic episodes (ST segment monitoring).Some teams use intra-operative EEG neurological monitoring to detect possible neurological deterioration during the operation.

2- General anaesthesia :

General anaesthesia has long been used in carotid surgery. Its main advantage lies in the improvement in cerebral tolerance to temporary ischaemia caused by carotid clamping, achieved by rapid-elimination anaesthetic agents.It also reduces cerebral metabolism, offers better myocardial protection and creates a degree of comfort for the doctor. Furthermore, this technique poses the dual problem of intra-operative haemodynamic balance and neurological monitoring during the arterial clamping period.

3- Loco-regional anaesthesia :

Historically, the first carotid thromboendarterectomy under locoregional anaesthesia was performed in 1953 (57).But this technique was abandoned at the time, as general anaesthetic techniques were developed, which gave the impression of obtaining better cerebral protection during the clamping period. Nevertheless, from the 1970s onwards, many teams re-adopted loco-regional anaesthesia as the technique offering the best neurological monitoring by cerebral monitoring during carotid clamping on an awake patient.Thanks to strict monitoring of the neurological state during the clamping period, the use of a carotid shunt was much less frequent: 4 to 6% in the case of unilateral stenosis, 10 to 20% in the presence of an occlusion of the contralateral internal carotid artery (58).Loco-regional anaesthesia also means that the patient can get up early, at a lower cost and with a shorter hospital stay.However, this technique is not without its disadvantages, particularly in relation to the puncture zone, which can easily cause nerve and vascular damage. The anaesthetic may also be toxic to the arteries (59).

X-SURGICAL TECHNIQUES

1- Approach :

The most traditional and widely used approach is the pre-sterno-cleido-mastoid cervicotomy.

2- Revascularisation techniques :

There are currently three surgical techniques for revascularisation of the internal carotid artery (ICA) in current practice: (60)

✓ Open carotid endarterectomy with longitudinal arteriotomy.
✓ Eversion carotid endarterectomies, which require sectioning of the ICA or the primitive common artery.
✓ Venous or prosthetic bypasses.

3- Open endarterectomy :

This is the technique most frequently used in carotid surgery. After making a vertical incision in the neck, the surgeon will dissect the carotid artery to remove the atherosclerotic plaque. He then proceeds to close the artery, using one of two methods: either directly by suturing, or suturing over a patch to widen the artery (Figure 14).

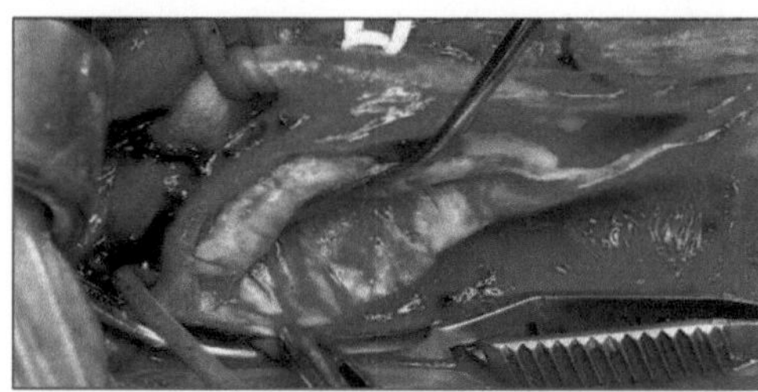

Figure 14: Open endarterectomy technique.

The enlargement patch is recommended to offset the risk of restenosis (61).This patch can be venous or prosthetic, and has the advantage over direct closure of not narrowing the arterial lumen and of reducing haemodynamic disturbances so as to reduce myointimal hyperplasia.Consequently, the use of patches reduces restenosis and homolateral stroke due to thrombosis (62).In a prospective randomised study by Aburahma (63), the rate of early homolateral disabling stroke after direct suture was higher than after patch closure (4.4% versus 0.4% respectively).

In contrast to this study, the NASCET results showed no significant differences between direct and patch closure (64).Systematic use of the patch is not always recommended.It would be preferable to use this technique only as a preventive measure in small carotid arteries or when the arteriotomy extends beyond the carotid bulb (5).

In this respect, Archie (5) has shown from a study of 1360 endarterectomies that patch closure is highly recommended in cases where the arteriotomy extends well beyond the carotid bulb. The venous patch is the best closure material, provided that the vein diameter is greater than 3.5 mm.

4- Eversion endarterectomy :

The surgical technique consists of eversion by transection of the internal carotid artery at its origin, or more rarely the primary carotid artery 10 to 20 mm distal to the bifurcation, followed by reimplantation by terminolateral anastomosis in the first case or termino-terminal anastomosis in the second case (Figure 15).

This technique can also be performed by sectioning the internal carotid artery downstream of the stenotic lesion and performing a longitudinal arteriotomy straddling the primary carotid artery (Chevalier technique).

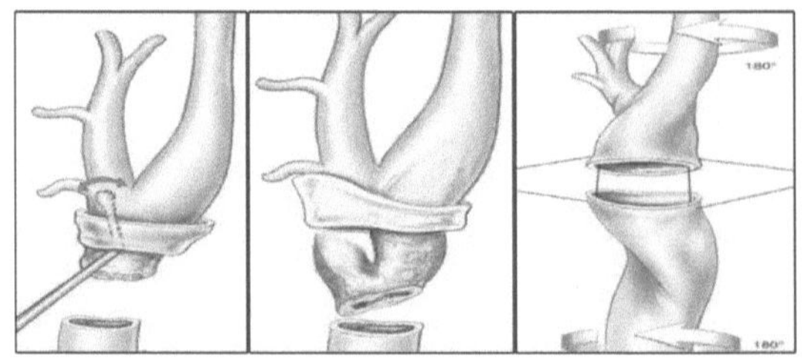

Figure 15: Eversion endarterectomy technique (65).

Endarterectomy by eversion offers the advantage of perfect control of the distal plaque and the absence of prosthetic material. It is particularly indicated in cases of longitudinally extensive plaque on the internal carotid artery. The main disadvantage of this method is the extensive arterial dissection, which can lead to increased peripheral nerve morbidity and frequent repeat surgery for post-operative haematoma. It also has the disadvantage of being more technically complex. Several studies have been carried out to compare the cost-effectiveness of the two techniques: conventional endarterectomy and eversion endarterectomy. The authors consider that conventional endarterectomy remains the gold standard, despite the advantages of the eversion technique (65).

5- Carotid bypass :

The principle of this method consists of a termino-lateral anastomosis on the primary carotid artery in a healthy area, followed by a termino-lateral anastomosis on the internal carotid artery downstream of the stenotic lesions (Figure 16).

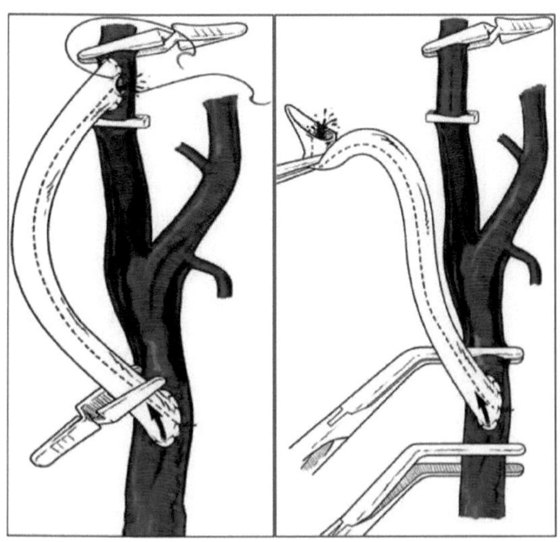

Figure 16: Carotid artery bypass graft using PTFE (66).

This technique is electively indicated when atheromatous lesions ascend on the internal carotid artery or descend on the primary carotid artery, thus avoiding an excessively long endarterectomy zone and distal plaque stoppages (67). In a study by Voirin et al (68), the cumulative morbidity and mortality rate (CMR) of the surgical team after carotid bypass surgery was 1.6% for a population of 185 patients. This CMR was relatively low, concluding that bypass surgery could be a good alternative to endarterectomy.

XI- MECHANISMS OF NEUROLOGICAL ACCIDENTS DURING CAROTID SURGERY

The most significant postoperative risk, and the one that determines the cumulative morbidity and mortality rate, is that of neurological strokes, which are often disabling. These neurological accidents can be caused by three main mechanisms:

1- Embolic mechanism :

These are emboli of atheromatous, cruoric or gaseous material which occur after the declamping manoeuvre or during dissection of the carotid bulb, particularly in the case of an ulcerated plaque.

2- Hemodynamic mechanism :

These accidents may be secondary: either to a reduction in regional cerebral blood flow during clamping, following ineffective collateralisation or intraoperative hypotension (69); or to rarer revascularisation accidents caused by possibly reversible reperfusion oedema or cerebral haemorrhage with a more serious prognosis.

3- Thrombotic mechanism :

In this case, the neurological accident is related to a technical fault in the endarterectomy procedure. Prevention involves visualising the end of the plaque to ensure that it is perfectly attached to the arterial wall.

XII- CEREBRAL PROTECTION

The benefits of carotid surgery are considered to be optimal when the neurological events that can occur during the perioperative period are prevented.

Cerebral protection during carotid surgery is therefore essential. It is provided by pharmacological and non-pharmacological means, and by the use of a shunt.

1- Pharmacological means :

The aim of pharmacological means is to induce a decrease in cellular metabolic activity during cerebral hypoperfusion. Heparinisation is essential to ensure adequate anticoagulation during clamping, thus avoiding distal intracerebral thrombosis.

2- Non-pharmacological means :

Cerebral protection requires good haemodynamic stability during the operation, limiting hyper- and hypotensive episodes.Hypotensive attacks result in hypo-cerebral flow due to a reduction in perfusion pressure. This can lead to cerebral ischaemic accidents. Arterial pressure must be increased during carotid clamping to ensure good collateral support. Cerebral protection also requires perfect oxygenation of brain tissue, with the aim of achieving optimum oxygen saturation (99 to 100%). Normo-capnia is also essential.

3- Use of a shunt during carotid surgery :

The shunt is a polyethylene tube placed in the carotid lumen through the arteriotomy. It can be short or long, with olives or balloons. It is important to exclude narrow-gauge shunts < 3 mm, which are generally associated with thrombosis (Figure 17).

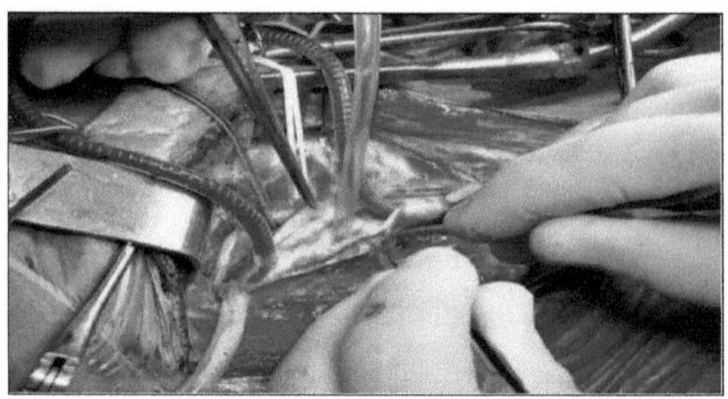

Figure 17: Fitting the shunt.

The purpose of the shunt is to maintain anterograde cerebral flow in the carotid axis during clamping. Its installation theoretically eliminates any cerebral ischaemia that may occur at this time (70). Several series have demonstrated that the shunt can normalise a disturbed EEG after clamping (71). Shunts may give rise to complications of their own, including cerebral embolisms (gaseous, cruoric, atheromatous, etc.), traumatic intimal lesions and dissection or perforation of the internal carotid artery during shunt insertion or extraction. In addition, performing endarterectomy with a shunt creates an additional technical difficulty for the surgeon.

<h1 style="text-align:center">XIII- RESULTS</h1>

1- Early operative mortality :

Table III summarises the mortality rates of certain series in the literature.

Table III: Mortality rates following carotid surgery :

Authors	Number of patients	Operative mortality rate (%)
Archie (5)	1360	1
Ohara (6)	3360	0,5
P Garvin (7)	2331	0,7
M Meller (8)	718	0,2
Sun J (9)	547	0,2

2- Early complications :

2-1- Neurological complications :

2-1-1- Central neurological complications :

The main operative risk in carotid surgery is central neurological complications, the mechanisms of which may be, as previously described: (72)

✓ **Embolic :**

Cerebral embolism is the cause of one third of post-operative neurological complications (73). Mobilisation of the carotid bifurcation prior to clamping, the presence of residual flaps at the thromboendarterectomy site and the formation of platelet aggregates on a stenosing suture are all potential sources of emboli destined for the brain.

✓ Intolerance to clamping :

Intolerance of clamping is the second most common cause of post-operative neurological complications. The hypoflow induced by clamping causes variable cerebral suffering, which is reversible in the majority of cases when ischaemic areas are reperfused.

✓ Thrombotic :

Thrombosis of the internal carotid artery is the third most common cause of post-operative neurological complications. A technical error is often the cause of this occlusion. The most frequent technical faults are intimal detachment in the area where the thromboendarterectomy is stopped, and the use of sutures which cause stenoses (74). It is essential to diagnose these by CT or MRI.

✓ Revascularisation oedema :

Revascularisation oedema is often suspected in the presence of unilateral headaches, convulsions or altered consciousness. It is diagnosed by a brain scan. This oedema is often regressive, but it can lead to a dreadful complication: cerebral haemorrhage, which is often serious.

Its management is based on anti-oedematous treatment combined with the maintenance of stable haemodynamics.

2-1-2- Neurological complications due to damage to the pairs cranial :

In almost 2/3 of cases, peripheral nerve damage is transient and very rarely life-threatening. Nerve damage may be transient or permanent, depending on the mechanism. Lesions caused by traction, compression, electrocoagulation, clamping and haematoma usually regenerate in a few weeks to two months, whereas lesions caused by ligature or section are permanent.

The incidence of these local neurological lesions varies between 5 and 80% depending on the type of study and the diagnostic methods used (75).

2-2- Hemodynamic complications :

Haemodynamic stability during carotid surgery is very important, both during and after the operation, and both hyper- and hypotension must be avoided.The aim is to maintain a stable pressure level, as a sufficiently sustained drop in local perfusion pressure can render tolerance mechanisms vulnerable and ineffective.

Arterial hypertension is also common, with a particularly high risk in the first 48 hours after surgery (76).Hypertension is associated with a risk of death, stroke and myocardial ischaemia in patients who often have coronary artery disease. It is treated with short half-life anti-hypertensives such as nicardipine, beta-blockers and urapidil.

2-3- Cardiac complications :

Cardiac morbidity, essentially myocardial ischaemia, occurs mainly in patients with known coronary disease. This justifies close monitoring of patients at risk, with repeated ECGs and cardiac enzyme assays.

2-4- Cervical haematomas :

Hypertensive attacks can cause haemorrhage at arterial sutures and lead to haematomas (62). These haematomas may also be caused by incorrect haemostasis, or leakage from the suture line facilitated by an overdose of heparin. Cervical haematomas are considered as frequent post-operative complications. In the literature, their frequency varies from 0.7% to 5.5% (5, 77). There are two types of haematoma: subcutaneous haematoma, which does not require repeat surgery, and compressive haematoma, which deviates from the trachea and requires emergency surgery.

3- Late complications :

These are mainly restenosis and late thrombosis, which can take a variable amount of time to appear.

3-1- Late restenosis :

Restenosis is defined as a reduction in the arterial lumen of the internal carotid artery $\geq 50\%$. The incidence of restenosis $> 50\%$ varies from 5 to 36% (78).

There are two types of restenosis:
✓ Early restenosis: this occurs within a year of endarterectomy and is most likely to be caused by intimal hyperplasia. In this case, surgical management is unusual.

✓ Late restenosis: detected after 24 months. They are often of atheromatous origin and have an emboligenic potential close to that of the atheromatous lesion initially treated. Surgery should be considered in these cases (79).

For Ballard (80), in a series of 1488 endarterectomies, the rate of restenosis was 2% at 5 years, 3% at 10 years and 3.5% at 15 years.In the Crest study (81), the rate of restenosis was estimated at 6% at 2 years. Ohara (6) reported on a series of 201 reoperations for carotid restenosis, 175 of which were atherosclerotic and 26 caused by myointimal hyperplasia. Angioplasty appears to be an interesting alternative for the treatment of late restenosis (82). The surgical management of restenosis is tricky because the surgical approach is made through scar tissue, with a risk of vascular effraction and damage to the cranial nerves (83).

3-2- Late thrombosis :

These are late complications that can go unnoticed or lead to a stroke. The time to onset varies. They can be early, with a fibrinocrust thrombus on contact with a patch, or late, with the completion of a restenosis process.

XIV- MDCT IN CAROTID SURGERY

The cumulative morbidity-mortality rate (CMMR) assessed at 30 days post-operatively, consists of the sum of neurological cerebral accidents (TIA or stroke), major cardiological events and deaths.

Table IV: Comparison of the MDCT of certain published series.

Author	Number of patients	TCMM
Archie (5)	1360	1,5%
ECST (41)	3026	7,4%
Rockman (84)	2476	2,4%

A number of risk factors predictive of early mortality have been mentioned in various studies, including: advanced age, female gender, diabetes, etc. and the existence of other sites of atherosclerosis. However, results vary from one study to another (85).

2- Early neurological complications :

Among the factors identified as predictive of early neurological complications, some were patient-related and others were technical. According to the literature, the use of a shunt, the absence of antithrombotic treatment and intraoperative blood pressure instability were associated with an increased operative risk (45).In the meta-analyses by Rothwell et al (86), the combined rates of stroke and death at 30 days were higher when the stenosis was symptomatic (5.1%) than when it was asymptomatic (3.3%).Eight factors have been identified as predictive of the risk of surgery, including: female gender, age over 75, systolic blood pressure > 180 mmHg, obliterative arterial disease of the lower limbs, cerebral rather than retinal vascular events, occlusion of the contralateral internal carotid artery, stenosis of the ipsilateral carotid siphon and stenosis of the ipsilateral external carotid artery (86).According to a multivariate analysis including the results of the ECST (39), four independent predictive factors were significant, summarised as follows: female gender, systolic blood pressure > 180 mm Hg, arteriopathy of the lower limbs and a cerebral rather than retinal event. Comparison of these results with those of NASCET (38) revealed two significant common risk factors for death and/or stroke at 30 days: a cerebral rather than retinal event and occlusion of the contralateral internal carotid artery. With regard to surgical techniques, several published studies (5, 87) emphasise the benefit of the patch in reducing ischaemic events following carotid surgery.

Comparative studies using different patches have been carried out. For Archie (5), in a series of 1360 endarterectomies, systematic use of the patch reduced the risk of ischaemic accidents to around 1.3%. The same study suggests that these accidents are more frequent after closure with a Dacron patch (1.7%) compared with closure with a venous patch (0.3%).

3- Late restenosis :

Several series (5, 80, 87, 88) have demonstrated that patch closure reduces the risk of late restenosis compared with direct closure.From a technical point of view, some studies have found that eversion endarterectomy is less likely to result in late restenosis than the conventional technique (89). Other studies (26), comparing eversion endarterectomy with "open" endarterectomy, concluded that there was no difference between these two methods in terms of the percentage of restenosis.The risk of restenosis after endarterectomy is also greater in women and when the diameter of the internal carotid artery is < 4 mm (64).

XVI- ANGIOPLASTY OF THE INTERNAL CAROTID ARTERY

1- Indications:

According to the latest recommendations from the French National Authority for Health (HAS), angioplasty of the internal carotid artery is only suitable for certain patients.

The inclusion criteria were as follows:

✓ A patient with a hostile neck.

✓ A patient with radial stenosis.

✓ The case of a restenosis restenosis when a revascularisation revascularisation is indicated.

The indications for angioplasty of the internal carotid artery, as an alternative to surgery, are elucidated as follows: (Figures 18 and 19)

✓ In asymptomatic patients :

o Carotid angioplasty should be considered for patients with stenoses between 60 and 99%, with a high surgical risk and in the presence of imaging criteria predictive of an ipsilateral stroke risk, provided that the patient's life expectancy exceeds five years and that the risk of stroke or death at 30 days is < 3%.

o In symptomatic patients :

o Angioplasty may be an alternative to surgery if symptoms are less than 6 months old in patients under 70, provided that the risk of stroke or death at 30 days is <6%.

Recommendation 19		
Carotid stenting may be considered in selected asymptomatic patients who have been deemed by the multidisciplinary team to be "high-risk for surgery" and who have an asymptomatic 60—99% stenosis in the presence of one or more imaging characteristics that may be associated with an increased risk of late ipsilateral stroke,[e] provided documented procedural risks are <3% and the patient's life expectancy exceeds 5 years	IIb	B

Recommendation 38		
When revascularisation is indicated in patients who have suffered carotid territory symptoms within the preceding 6 months and who are aged <70 years, carotid stenting may be considered an alternative to endarterectomy, provided the documented procedural death/stroke rate is <6%	IIb	A

Figures 18 and 19: European recommendations for carotid stenting in asymptomatic patients (21).

2- Technical aspects :

Endoluminal carotid angioplasty involves puncturing the femoral artery in the groin and inserting a dilatation balloon combined with a stent (metal spring) (Figure 20).

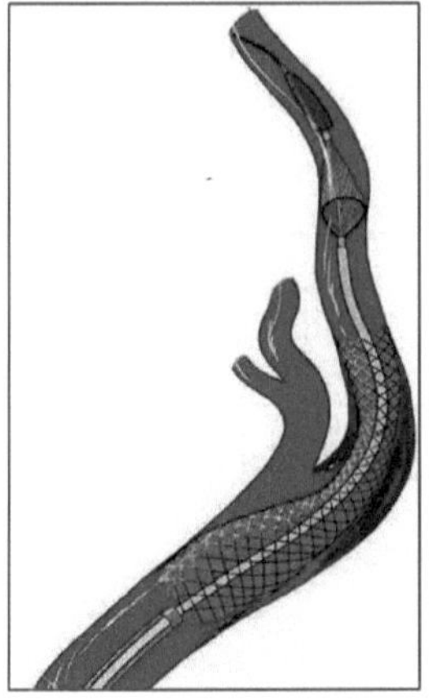

Figure 20: Carotid stenting (66).

3- Advantages :

The advantages of this technique are its simplicity and rapidity, the reduction in carotid clamping time to the time required for balloon inflation, and the absence of a surgical approach.

4- Complications :

4-1- Neurological complications :

This is the major risk of this procedure. The onset of ischaemic stroke in the downstream territory can have several mechanisms:

- Distal embolisms.

- Occlusion of the internal carotid artery after dilatation due to spasm, dissection or thrombosis of the dilated site or stent.

4-2- Technical complications :

These complications include

- Catheterisation failures.
- The complications of catheterization :embolisms of dissection, perforation.

- Complications at the puncture site.

- Residual post-dilation stenosis.

4-3- Restenosis :

Angioplasty causes myointimal hyperplasia, which is a source of early restenosis.

XVII-CONCLUSION

Atherosclerotic stenosis of the internal carotid artery is a frequent and serious condition, with a high risk of ischaemic neurological events, often severe, occurring homolaterally to the stenosis. They are diagnosed by non-invasive investigations, and are always amenable to optimal medical treatment, combined in some cases with surgery.The indications for surgery are based on two key factors: the degree of stenosis and whether it is symptomatic or asymptomatic. These indications are now well codified, thanks to major randomised trials which have demonstrated the vital role of surgical treatment in improving the prognosis of carotid stenosis, taking into account the cumulative morbidity-mortality rate (CMMR) of the surgical team.There are various surgical techniques. Open carotid thromboendarterectomy with direct or patch closure is considered to be the technique of choice.Despite recent advances in interventional catheterisation, which have attempted to introduce percutaneous angioplasty with or without a stent into the therapeutic armoury for carotid atheromatosis, carotid endarterectomy remains the reference method for treating atheromatous carotid stenosis. The best treatment is still primary prevention of the risk factors for atherosclerosis, in particular tobacco control, as well as control of hypertension, diabetes and dyslipidaemia.

BIBLIOGRAPHY

1. Bruder N, Boussen S. Ischaemic stroke. Anesth Réanimation. 1 Jan 2017;3(1):25-36.

2. Saini V, Guada L, Yavagal DR. Global Epidemiology of Stroke and Access to Acute Ischemic Stroke Interventions. Neurology. 16 Nov 2021;97(20 Suppl 2): S6-16.

3. Adams HP, Bendixen BH, Kappelle LJ, Biller J, Love BB, Gordon DL, et al. Classification of subtype of acute ischemic stroke. Definitions for use in a multicenter clinical trial. TOAST. Trial of Org 10172 in Acute Stroke Treatment. Stroke. Jan 1993;24(1):35-41.

4. Rubio F, Martínez-Yélamos S, Cardona P, Krupinski J. Carotid endarterectomy: is it still a gold standard? Cerebrovasc Dis Basel Switz. 2005;20 Suppl 2:119-22.

5. Archie JP. A fifteen-year experience with carotid endarterectomy after a formal operative protocol requiring highly frequent patch angioplasty. J Vasc Surg. Apr 2000;31(4):724-35.

6. O'Hara PJ, Hertzer NR, Mascha EJ, Krajewski LP, Clair DG, Ouriel K. A prospective, randomized study of saphenous vein patching versus synthetic patching during carotid endarterectomy. J Vasc Surg. Feb 2002;35(2):324-32.

7. Garvin RP, Ryer EJ, Berger AL, Elmore JR. Long-term comparative effectiveness of carotid stenting versus carotid endarterectomy in a large tertiary care vascular surgery practice. J Vasc Surg. Oct 2018;68(4):1039-46.

8. Meller SM, Salim Al-Damluji M, Gutierrez A, Stilp E, Mena-Hurtado C. Carotid stenting versus endarterectomy for the treatment of carotid artery stenosis: Contemporary results from a large single center study. Catheter Cardiovasc Interv Off J Soc Card Angiogr Interv. Nov 2016;88(5):822-30.

9. Sun WJ, Gao FL, Qi XC, Wang YR, Peng DQ, Wu C, et al. [A single center large cohort study on perioperative complications of carotid endarterectomy of 547 cases]. Zhonghua Yi Xue Za Zhi. August 7, 2018;98(29):2331-5.

10. Mahmood SS, Levy D, Vasan RS, Wang TJ. The Framingham Heart Study and the Epidemiology of Cardiovascular Diseases: A Historical Perspective. Lancet. 15 March 2014;383(9921):999-1008.

11. De Courson H, Renou P. Hypertension and stroke. Anesth Réanimation. 1 Sep 2023;9(4):382-7.

12. Ai M. [Atherosclerosis (hypertension)]. Nihon Rinsho Jpn J Clin Med. May 2012;70(5):840-5.

13. Brownlee M. Lilly Lecture 1993. Glycation and diabetic complications. Diabetes. June 1994;43(6):836-41.

14. Leutenegger M, Bertin E. Diabetes mellitus and atherosclerosis. Physiopathology of diabetic macroangiopathy. Rev Médecine Interne. 1 Jan 1995;16(1):31-42.

15. Veyssier Belot C. [Tobacco smoking and cardiovascular risk]. Rev Med Interne. 1997;18(9):702-8.

16. Hurtubise J, McLellan K, Durr K, Onasanya O, Nwabuko D, Ndisang JF. The Different Facets of Dyslipidemia and Hypertension in Atherosclerosis. Curr Atheroscler Rep. Dec 2016;18(12):82.

17. Byington RP, Furberg CD, Crouse JR, Espeland MA, Bond MG. Pravastatin, Lipids, and Atherosclerosis in the Carotid Arteries (PLAC-II). Am J Cardiol. 28 Sep 1995;76(9):54C-59C.

18. Gokaldas R, Singh M, Lal S, Benenstein RJ, Sahni R. Carotid stenosis: from diagnosis to management, where do we stand? Curr Atheroscler Rep. 2015;17(2):480.

19. Carreira M, Duarte-Gamas L, Rocha-Neves J, Andrade JP, Fernando-Teixeira J. Management of The Carotid Artery Stenosis in Asymptomatic Patients. Rev Port Cir Cardio-Torac E Vasc Orgao Of Soc Port Cir Cardio-Torac E Vasc. 2020;27(3):159-66.

20. Pujia A, Rubba P, Spencer MP. Prevalence of extracranial carotid artery disease detectable by echo-Doppler in an elderly population. Stroke. June 1992;23(6):818-22.

21. Aboyans V, Ricco JB, Bartelink MLEL, Björck M, Brodmann M, Cohnert T, et al. 2017 ESC Guidelines on the Diagnosis and Treatment of Peripheral Arterial Diseases, in collaboration with the European Society for Vascular Surgery (ESVS): Document covering atherosclerotic disease of extracranial carotid and vertebral, mesenteric, renal, upper and lower extremity arteriesEndorsed by: the European Stroke Organization (ESO)The Task Force for the Diagnosis and Treatment of Peripheral Arterial Diseases of the European Society of Cardiology (ESC) and of the European Society for Vascular Surgery (ESVS). Eur Heart J. March 1, 2018;39(9):763-816.

22. Trihan JE, Lanéelle D, Thollot C, Escure E, Belhadj-Chaidi R, Delicque J,et al. Evaluation and quantification of carotid stenosis by Doppler ultrasound. J Imag Diagn Interv. Sep 1, 2019;2(4):204-16.

23. Grotta JC. Carotid Stenosis. Solomon CG, editor. N Engl J Med. Sep 19, 2013;369(12):1143-50.

24. Padayachee TS, Cox TC, Modaresi KB, Colchester AC, Taylor PR. The measurement of internal carotid artery stenosis: comparison of duplex with digital subtraction angiography. Eur J Vasc Endovasc Surg Off J Eur Soc Vasc Surg. Feb 1997;13(2):180-5.

25. Baqué J, Azarine A, Beyssen B, Bonneville JF, Cattin F, Long A. [Imaging of the extracranial carotid arteries: when, how and why?] J Radiol. June

2004;85(6 Pt 2):825-44.

26. Cao P, Giordano G, De Rango P, Zannetti S, Chiesa R, Coppi G, et al. Eversion versus conventional carotid endarterectomy: late results of a prospective multicenter randomized trial. J Vasc Surg. Jan 2000;31(1 Pt 1):19-30.

27. Kappelle LJ, Eliasziw M, Fox AJ, Sharpe BL, Barnett HJ. Importance of intracranial atherosclerotic disease in patients with symptomatic stenosis of the internal carotid artery. The North American Symptomatic Carotid Endarterectomy Trail. Stroke. Feb 1999;30(2):282-6.

28. Déglise S, Dubuis C, Mosimann P, Saucy F, Engelberger S, Hirt L, et al [Management of the carotid artery stenosis]. Rev Med Suisse. 19 June 2013;9(391):1305-11.

29. Mortele KJ, McTavish J, Ros PR. Current techniques of computed tomography. Helical CT, multidetector CT, and 3D reconstruction. Clin Liver Dis. Feb 2002;6(1):29-52.

30. Wardlaw J, Chappell F, Best J, Wartolowska K, Berry E. Non-invasive imaging compared with intra-arterial angiography in the diagnosis of symptomatic carotid stenosis: a meta-analysis. The Lancet. May 2006;367(9521):1503-12.

31. Long A, Lepoutre A, Corbillon E, Branchereau A. Critical review of non- or minimally invasive methods (duplex ultrasonography, MR- and CT-angiography) for evaluating stenosis of the proximal internal carotid artery. Eur J Vasc Endovasc Surg Off J Eur Soc Vasc Surg. July 2002;24(1):43-52.

32. Tarjàn Z, Pozzi Mucelli F, Frezza F, Pozzi Mucelli R. Three-dimensional reconstructions of carotid bifurcation from CT images: evaluation of different rendering methods. Eur Radiol. 1996;6(3):326-33.

33. Baqué J, Azarine A, Beyssen B, Bonneville JF, Cattin F, Long A. When, how and why should extracranial carotid artery imaging be performed? J Radiol. 1 June 2004;85(6, Part 2):825-44.

34. Serfaty JM, Chirossel P, Chevallier JM, Ecochard R, Froment JC, Douek PC. Accuracy of three-dimensional gadolinium-enhanced MR angiography in the assessment of extracranial carotid artery disease. AJR Am J Roentgenol. August 2000;175(2):455-63.

35. Yuan C, Mitsumori LM, Beach KW, Maravilla KR. Carotid atherosclerotic plaque: noninvasive MR characterization and identification of vulnerable lesions. Radiology. Nov 2001;221(2):285-99.

36. Boussel L, Serusclat A, Skilton M, Vincent F, Bernard S, Moulin P, et al. CV-WS-35 Reliability of carotid wall thickness measurement in high-resolution MRI. J Radiol. 1 Oct 2007;88(10):1526.

37. Rodriguez-Régent C, Naggara O, Beyssen B, Trystram D, Mas JL, Meder JF. Diagnosis of carotid stenosis. Arch Mal Coeur Vaiss - Prat. 1 Dec 2012;2012(213):9-12.

38. Ferguson GG, Eliasziw M, Barr HW, Clagett GP, Barnes RW, Wallace MC, et al. The North American Symptomatic Carotid Endarterectomy Trial: surgical results in 1415 patients. Stroke. Sept 1999;30(9):1751-8.

39. Randomised trial of endarterectomy for recently symptomatic carotid stenosis: final results of the MRC European Carotid Surgery Trial (ECST). Lancet Lond Engl. 9 May 1998;351(9113):1379-87.

40. Long A, Albertini JN, Muller S, Clément C. Conventional carotid artery surgery: a review of indications. J Neuroradiol. 1 June 2006;33(3):147-51.

41. Endarterectomy for asymptomatic carotid artery stenosis. Executive Committee for the Asymptomatic Carotid Atherosclerosis Study. JAMA. May

10, 1995;273(18):1421-8.

42. Habozit B. The silent brain infarct before and after carotid surgery. Ann Vasc Surg. Sept 1990;4(5):485-9.

43. Findlay JM, Marchak BE, Pelz DM, Feasby TE. Carotid endarterectomy: a review. Can J Neurol Sci J Can Sci Neurol. Feb 2004;31(1):22-36.

44. Barnett HJ, Taylor DW, Eliasziw M, Fox AJ, Ferguson GG, Haynes RB, et al. Benefit of carotid endarterectomy in patients with symptomatic moderate or severe stenosis. North American Symptomatic Carotid Endarterectomy Trial Collaborators. N Engl J Med. 12 Nov 1998;339(20):1415-25.

45. MRC European Carotid Surgery Trial: interim results for symptomatic patients with severe (70-99%) or with mild (0-29%) carotid stenosis. European Carotid Surgery Trialists' Collaborative Group. Lancet Lond Engl. 25 May 1991;337(8752):1235-43.

46. Endarterectomy for moderate symptomatic carotid stenosis: interim results from the MRC European Carotid Surgery Trial. Lancet Lond Engl. 8 June 1996;347(9015):1591-3.

47. Hertzer NR. The Current Status of Carotid Endarterectomy, Part I: Randomized Trials versus Medical Management. Ann Vasc Surg. August 2017;43:1-23.

48. Halliday A, Mansfield A, Marro J, Peto C, Peto R, Potter J, et al. Prevention of disabling and fatal strokes by successful carotid endarterectomy in patients without recent neurological symptoms: randomised controlled trial. Lancet Lond Engl. 8 May 2004;363(9420):1491-502.

49. Gladstone DJ, Oh J, Fang J, Lindsay P, Tu JV, Silver FL, et al. Urgency of carotid endarterectomy for secondary stroke prevention: results from the Registry of the Canadian Stroke Network. Stroke. August 2009;40(8):2776-82.

50. Giles MF, Rothwell PM. Risk of stroke early after transient ischaemic attack: a systematic review and meta-analysis. Lancet Neurol. Dec 2007;6(12):1063-72.

51. Rothwell PM, Eliasziw M, Gutnikov SA, Warlow CP, Barnett HJM, Carotid Endarterectomy Trialists Collaboration. Endarterectomy for symptomatic carotid stenosis in relation to clinical subgroups and timing of surgery. Lancet Lond Engl. 20 March 2004;363(9413):915-24.

52. Paty PSK, Darling RC, Feustel PJ, Bernardini GL, Mehta M, Ozsvath KJ, et al. Early carotid endarterectomy after acute stroke. J Vasc Surg. Jan 2004;39(1):148-54.

53. Fairhead JF, Rothwell PM. The need for urgency in identification and treatment of symptomatic carotid stenosis is already established. Cerebrovasc Dis Basel Switz. 2005;19(6):355-8.

54. Brandl R, Brauer RB, Maurer PC. Urgent carotid endarterectomy for stroke in evolution. VASA Z Gefasskrankheiten. May 2001;30(2):115-21.

55. Lindblad B, Persson NH, Takolander R, Bergqvist D. Does low-dose acetylsalicylic acid prevent stroke after carotid surgery? A double-blind, placebo- controlled randomized trial. Stroke. August 1993;24(8):1125-8.

56. Sadik JC, Riquier V, Koskas P, Zylberberg F, Beyloune-Mainardi C, Szmaragd V, et al. Transcranial Echo-Doppler: An update. J Radiol. July 2001;82(7):821-31.

57. Peitzman AB, Webster MW, Loubeau JM, Grundy BL, Bahnson HT. Carotid Endarterectomy under Regional (Conductive) Anesthesia: Ann Surg. July 1982;196(1):59-64.

58. Leseche G, Castier Y, Francis F, Besnard M. Optimisation of carotid endarterectomy results. J Mal Vasc. 1 May 2005;30(2):88-93.

59. Thermann F, Ukkat J, John E, Dralle H, Brauckhoff M. Frequency of transient ipsilateral vocal cord paralysis in patients undergoing carotid endarterectomy under local anaesthesia. J Vasc Surg. Jul 2007;46(1):37-40.

60. Garbé JF. Technical modalities of carotid endarterectomy. J Mal Vasc. 1 March 2016;41(2):108-9.

61. Counsell CE, Salinas R, Naylor R, Warlow CP. A systematic review of the randomised trials of carotid patch angioplasty in carotid endarterectomy. Eur J Vasc Endovasc Surg. Apr 1997;13(4):345-54.

62. Mannheim D, Weller B, Vahadim E, Karmeli R. Carotid endarterectomy with a polyurethane patch versus primary closure: a prospective randomized study. J Vasc Surg. March 2005;41(3):403-7; discussion 407-408.

63. AbuRahma AF, Khan JH, Robinson PA, Saiedy S, Short YS, Boland JP, et al. Prospective randomized trial of carotid endarterectomy with primary closure and patch angioplasty with saphenous vein, jugular vein, and polytetrafluoroethylene: perioperative (30-day) results. J Vasc Surg. Dec 1996;24(6):998-1006; discussion 1006-1007.

64. Golledge J, Cuming R, Davies AH, Greenhalgh RM. Outcome of selective patching following carotid endarterectomy. Eur J Vasc Endovasc Surg Off J Eur Soc Vasc Surg. May 1996;11(4):458-63.

65. Yasa H, Akyuz M, Yakut N, Aslan O, Akyuz D, Ozcem B, et al. Comparison of two surgical techniques for carotid endarterectomy: conventional and eversion. Neurosurgery. 2014;60(1-2):33-7.

66. Ricco JB, Marchand C, Neau JP, Marchand E, Cau J, Fébrer G. Prosthetic carotid bypass grafts for atherosclerotic lesions: a prospective study of 198 consecutive cases. Eur J Vasc Endovasc Surg Off J Eur Soc Vasc Surg. March 2009;37(3):272-8.

67. Irace L, Martinelli O, Stumpo R, Trenti E, Fornasin FR, Laurito A, et al

[Carotid-carotid bypass. Indications and results]. Minerva Cardioangiol. June 2003;51(3):329-35.

68. Voirin L, Magne JL, Farah I, Sessa C, Chichignoud B, Guidicelli H. [Carotid revascularizations by venous grafting: long-term results]. Chir Memoires Acad Chir. 1997;122(5-6):346-50.

69. Lawrence PF, Alves JC, Jicha D, Bhirangi K, Dobrin PB. Incidence, timing, and causes of cerebral ischemia during carotid endarterectomy with regional anesthesia. J Vasc Surg. Feb 1998;27(2):329-34; discussion 335-337.

70. Halsey JH. Risks and benefits of shunting in carotid endarterectomy. The International Transcranial Doppler Collaborators. Stroke. Nov 1992;23(11):1583-7.

71. Pinkerton JA. EEG as a criterion for shunt need in carotid endarterectomy. Ann Vasc Surg. Nov 2002;16(6):756-61.

72. Rothwell PM, Gutnikov SA, Warlow CP, European Carotid Surgery Trialist's Collaboration. Reanalysis of the final results of the European Carotid Surgery Trial. Stroke. Feb 2003;34(2):514-23.

73. De Borst GJ, Moll FL, van de Pavoordt HD, Mauser HW, Kelder JC, Ackerstaf RG. Stroke from carotid endarterectomy: when and how to reduce perioperative stroke rate? Eur J Vasc Endovasc Surg Off J Eur Soc Vasc Surg. June 2001;21(6):484-9.

74. Ross CB, Ranval TJ. Intraoperative use of stents for the management of unacceptable distal internal carotid artery end points during carotid endarterectomy: short-term and midterm results. J Vasc Surg. Sept 2000;32(3):420-7; 427-8.

75. Regina G, Angiletta D, Impedovo G, De Robertis G, Fiorella M, Carratu' MR. Dexamethasone minimizes the risk of cranial nerve injury during CEA. J Vasc Surg. Jan 2009;49(1):99-102; discussion 103.

76. Biller J, Feinberg WM, Castaldo JE, Whittemore AD, Harbaugh RE, Dempsey RJ, et al. Guidelines for carotid endarterectomy: a statement for healthcare professionals from a Special Writing Group of the Stroke Council, American Heart Association. Circulation. Feb 10, 1998;97(5):501-9.

77. North American Symptomatic Carotid Endarterectomy Trial Collaborators, Barnett HJM, Taylor DW, Haynes RB, Sackett DL, Peerless SJ, et al. Beneficial effect of carotid endarterectomy in symptomatic patients with high-grade carotid stenosis. N Engl J Med. August 15, 1991;325(7):445-53.

78. Kownator S. Ultrasound monitoring after carotid endarterectomy: a critical review. Ann Cardiol Angéiologie. Jan 2004;53(1):44-8.

79. O'Donnell TF, Rodriguez AA, Fortunato JE, Welch HJ, Mackey WC. Management of recurrent carotid stenosis: should asymptomatic lesions be treated surgically? J Vasc Surg. August 1996;24(2):207-12.

80. Ballard JL, Romano M, Abou-Zamzam AM, Teruya TH. Carotid artery patch angioplasty: impact and outcome. Ann Vasc Surg. Jan 2002;16(1):12-6.

81. Lal BK, Beach KW, Roubin GS, Lutsep HL, Moore WS, Malas MB, et al. Restenosis after carotid artery stenting and endarterectomy: a secondary analysis of CREST, a randomised controlled trial. Lancet Neurol. Sep 2012;11(9):755-63.

82. Gasparis AP, Ricotta L, Cuadra SA, Char DJ, Purtill WA, Van Bemmelen PS, et al. High-risk carotid endarterectomy: fact or fiction. J Vasc Surg. Jan 2003;37(1):40-6.

83. Ricco JB, Lemonnier T, Koskas F, Marchand C. Treatment of carotid stenosis: surgery, the gold standard. Presse Médicale. Sept 2004;33(16):1108-12.

84. Rockman CB, Castillo J, Adelman MA, Jacobowitz GR, Gagne PJ, Lamparello PJ, et al. Carotid endarterectomy in female patients: are the concerns

of the Asymptomatic Carotid Atherosclerosis Study valid? J Vasc Surg. Feb 2001;33(2):236-40; discussion 240-241.

85. Roubin GS, New G, Iyer SS, Vitek JJ, Al-Mubarak N, Liu MW, et al. Immediate and late clinical outcomes of carotid artery stenting in patients with symptomatic and asymptomatic carotid artery stenosis: a 5-year prospective analysis. Circulation. 30 Jan 2001;103(4):532-7.

86. Rothwell P m., Slattery J, Warlow C p. A Systematic Comparison of the Risks of Stroke and Death Due to Carotid Endarterectomy for Symptomatic and Asymptomatic Stenosis. Stroke. Feb 1996;27(2):266-9.

87. AbuRahma AF, Hannay RS, Khan JH, Robinson PA, Hudson JK, Davis EA. Prospective randomized study of carotid endarterectomy with polytetrafluoroethylene versus collagen-impregnated Dacron (Hemashield) patching: perioperative (30-day) results. J Vasc Surg. Jan 2002;35(1):125-30.

TABLE OF CONTENTS